AF264377

HUMANS: GUIDE TO HAIRSTYLE

BY

KEVEON E WHITLEY

Humans Guide to Hairstyling
Volume 1: Understanding the 12 Sections of The Human Head

First Edition
Published in the United States of America

ISBN: _______________ (Print)

Preface

Hello, my fellow human. My name is KevEon Whitley. I was born in St. Louis, Missouri, to Beverly, my mother & William, my father. As a child, I spent a few years in Alton, Illinois, but the majority of my childhood, youth, and adulthood was spent in St. Louis. In 2010, at 22, I decided to move to NYC, where I swiftly began my education in Cosmetology, which I completed in 2011.

Months later, I began working in a Salon. Then, soon after gained my license in Cosmetology & received my educator's license in Cosmetology in the State of New York in 2019. The information in this book has been within me growing & simplifying itself down to the simplest form, since I was a child and teenager, when I made poor attempts at cutting my own hair, and soon after, my friends and then clients behind the chair. I have seen the need for this knowledge to be widespread, as it connects us all in this very human experience. It is then that I realized that hair styling is a life skill and should be foundational in human skill sets.

This is my contribution to that confusion & the solution.

NOTE: The use of numbers is with intention and a reflection of numbers used in the universe.

Upon my entering cosmetology school, I received mannequins to practice on. We were starting our hairstyling phase & the instructor was going to conduct a blowout for the class. As the sectioned out their mannequin, I vividly recall myself asking the instructor, "How many sections of the head are there?"
They responded, "Well, it changes upon the service; there are many different section styles Hairstylists use & will go over."

In short, I never received my answer; however, I spent over 10 years behind the chair. I remembered I told myself I wanted to give back & teach at a cosmetology school. Upon hiring, educators receive a multitude of mannequins to work with & see 1st hand the learning complexities of all people. I was able to answer my very

complex question.
Only through my 10+ Years behind the chair & 2 years in education as
I able to make this breakthrough.

I developed a lesson to navigate the human head with ease, allowing
each region of the Head Care & Efficiency.

I learned there are three sections of the Head...
Crown: The top of your head.

Temporal Region, which is the largest of the head, moves across
the right side of the head (above ears) throughout the back towards
the left side of the head (above ears) & the Nape, which is the lower
region of the head.

Then I thought, how many points of the human head are there?

In haircutting, you learn that there is only one point & guideline for
the head... However, I am not referencing haircutting in this volume,
simply the human head.

So, to answer the question, how many points of the human head are
there.. the Answer is 12.

If separating into the three regions, at just the nape, you have 3 (with
strong consideration of the 2 points behind the ear, making it 5),
when combining the Nape & Temporal, you have 7, altogether there
are 12 points.

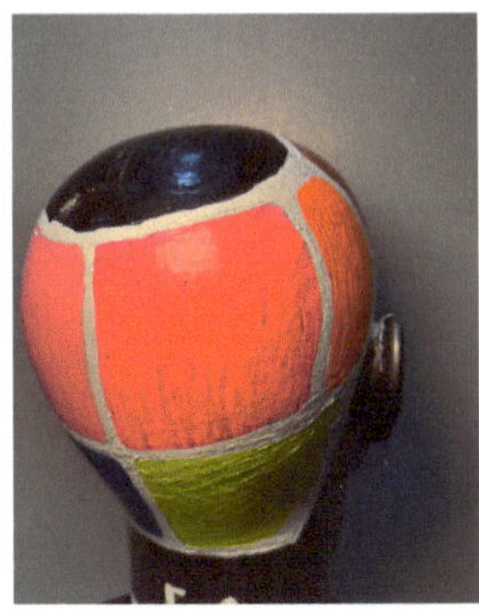
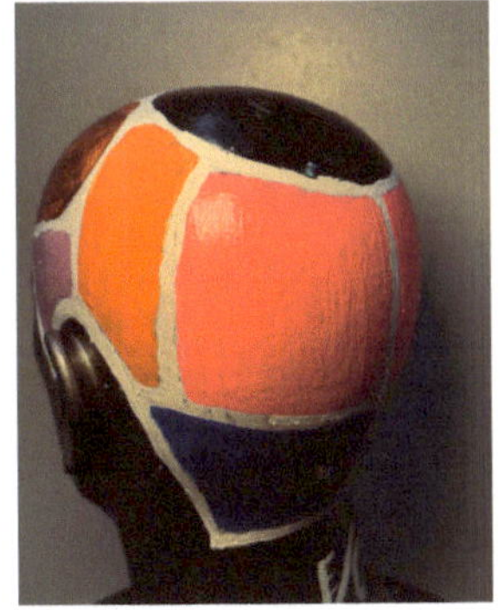
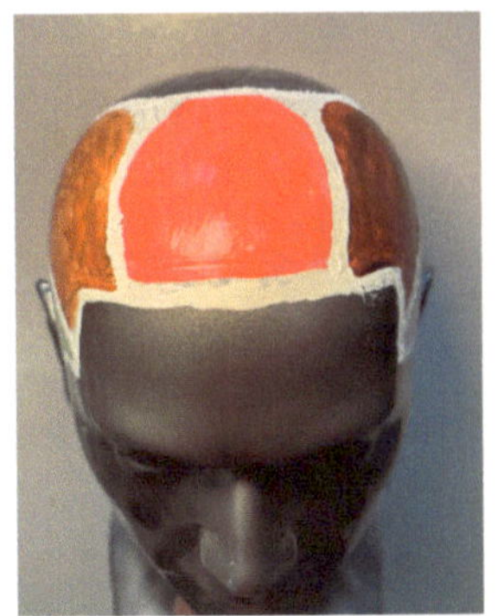

See the "Play" on #Numbers.

Now, truthfully, this message is effective for those with a buzz
cut because, in explaining the sections of the hair, I will also
explain where the hair lives in each section, which benefits scalp
manipulation & hair growth. However, I am sharing it in the hope
that it will help & guide users with ease as they grow their hair, while
also aiding in managing time.

Made with much consideration for stylists/hair magicians globally.
Fear not, human hairstyling will forever be a profitable skill with the
help of an expert.t

TABLE OF CONTENT

NAPE LEFT

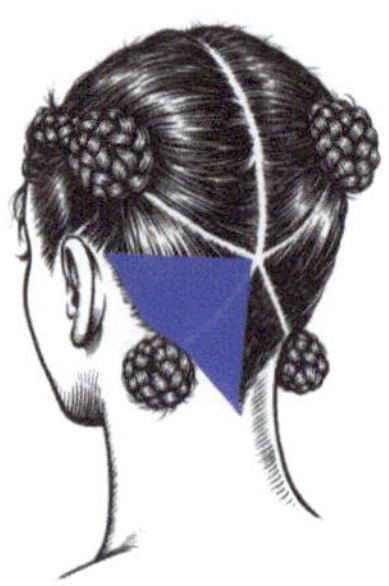

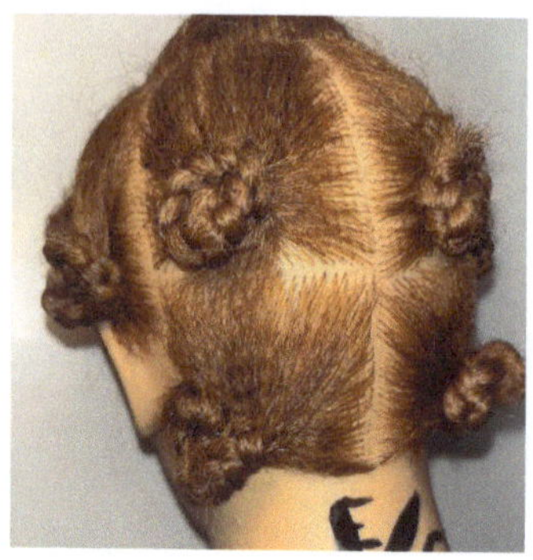
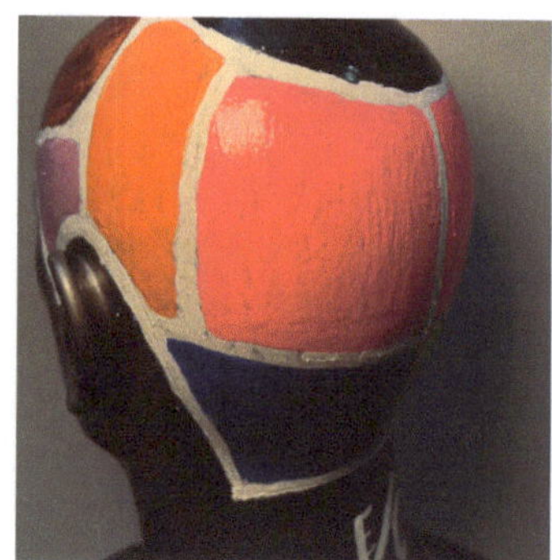

The **Nape Left Region** outlines the lower perimeter of the hairline beneath the occipital bone, forming the base curve of the head. Hair in this region covers the center of the neck and extends slightly toward the corners, moving downward in a subtle diagonal direction toward the face.

When performing Scalp Manipulation, Detangling & Hairstyling, position and guide the hair downward in a slightly diagonal direction toward the face.

NAPE RIGHT

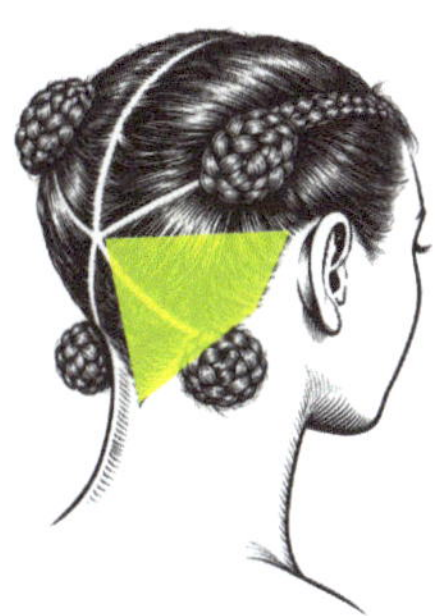

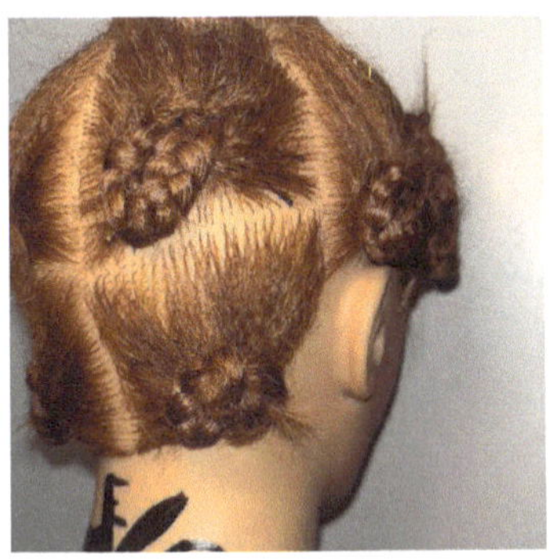
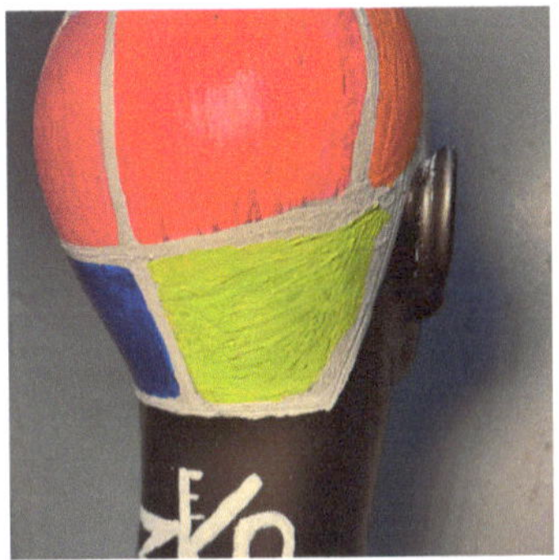

The **Nape Right Region** outlines the lower perimeter of the hairline beneath the occipital bone, forming the base curve of the head. Hair in this region covers the center of the neck and extends slightly toward the corners, moving downward in a subtle diagonal direction toward the face.

When performing Scalp Manipulation, Detangling, or Hairstyling, position and guide the hair downward in a slightly diagonal direction toward the face.

TEMPORAL LEFT

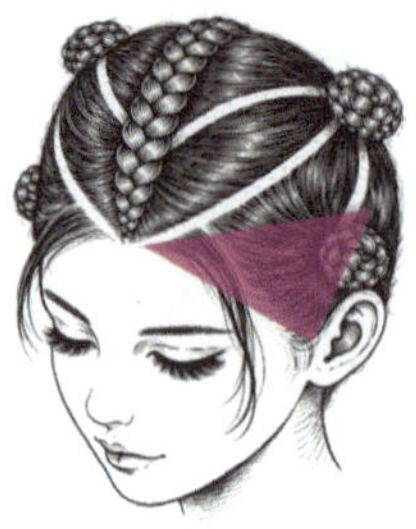

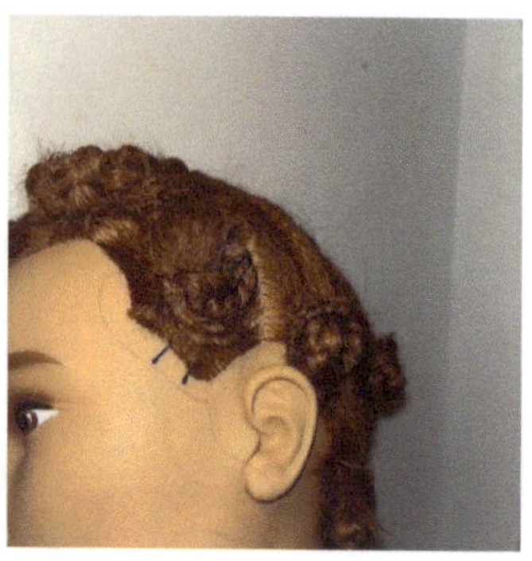
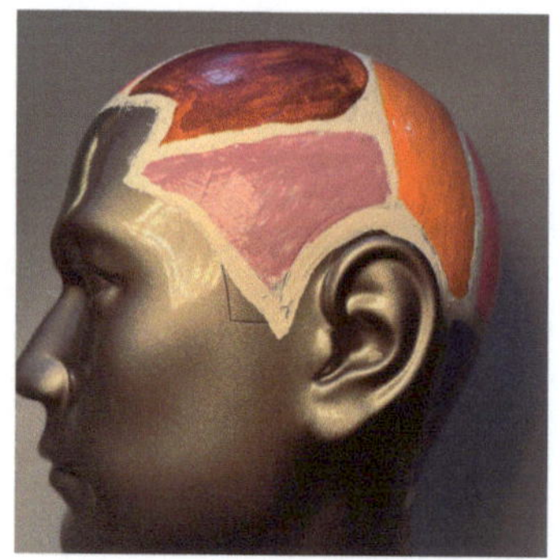

The **Temporal Region** is located at the upper side of the ear, outlining the outer perimeter of the hairline from the sideburn into the rounded "C" shape that frames the face. Hair in this region connects the back of the head to the face and naturally moves forward rather than downward or backward.

When performing Scalp Manipulation, Detangling, or Hairstyling, position and guide the hair in a forward motion toward the face.

TEMPORAL RIGHT

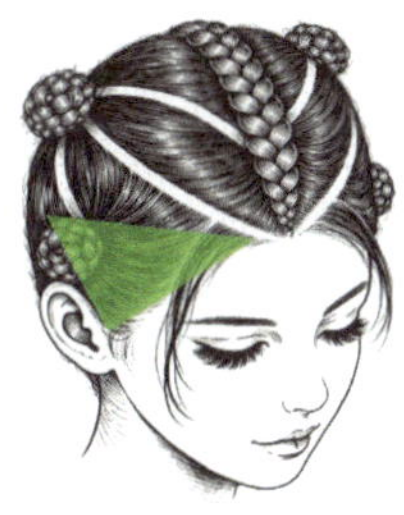

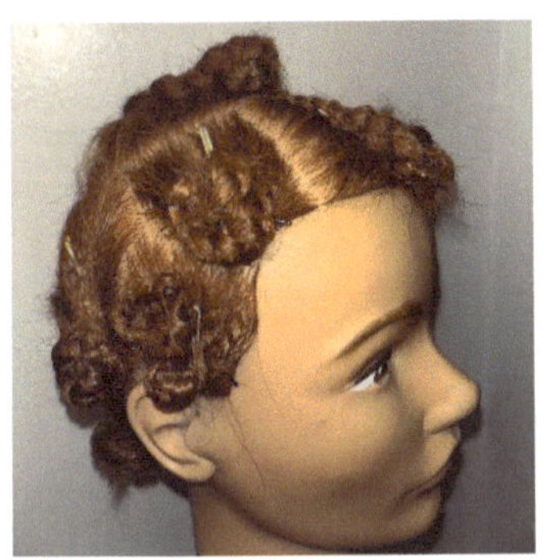
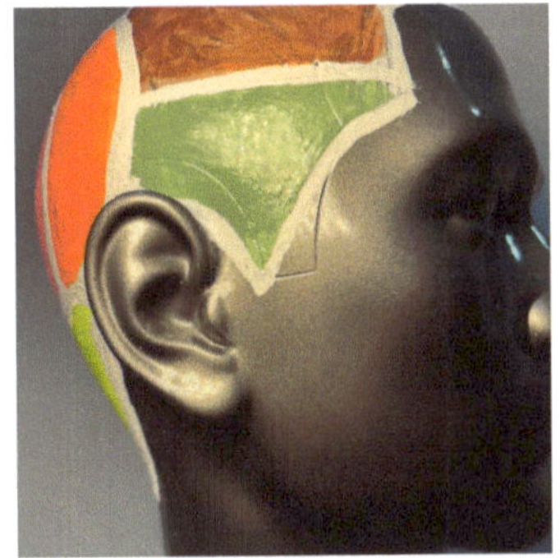

The **Temporal Region** is located at the upper side of the ear, outlining the outer perimeter of the hairline from the sideburn into the rounded "C" shape that frames the face. Hair in this region connects the back of the head to the face and naturally moves forward rather than downward or backward.

When performing Scalp Manipulation, Detangling, or Hairstyling, position and guide the hair in a forward motion toward the face.

BACK LEFT

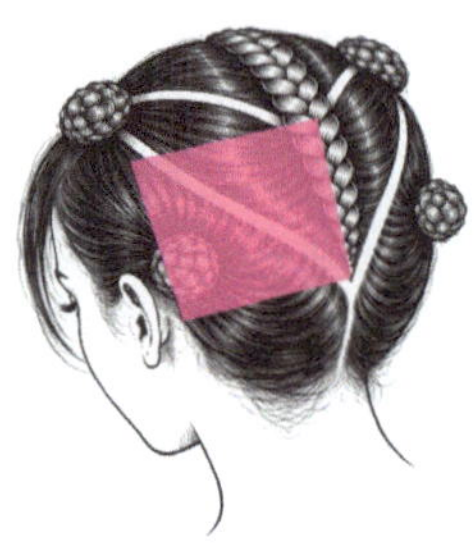

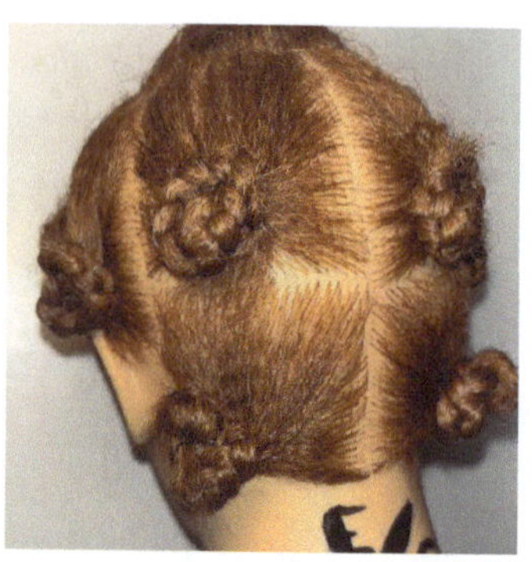
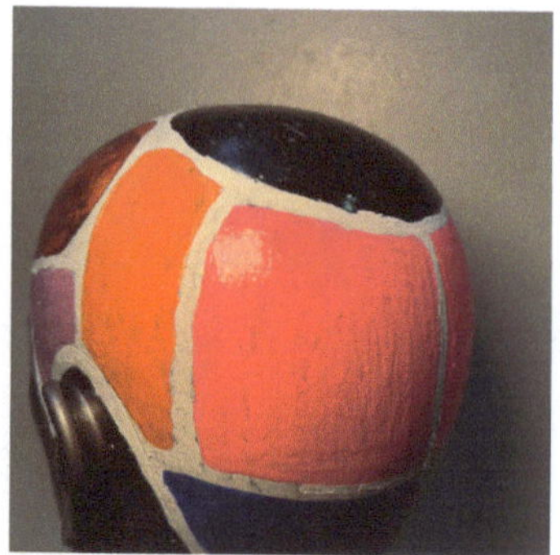

The **Back Left Region** outlines the space above the occipital bone and includes the visible upper back portion of the head. Hair in this region covers the neck and naturally falls straight downward, aligning with the spine.

When performing Scalp Manipulation, Detangling & Hairstyling, position and guide the hair downward toward the center in alignment with the spine.

BACK RIGHT

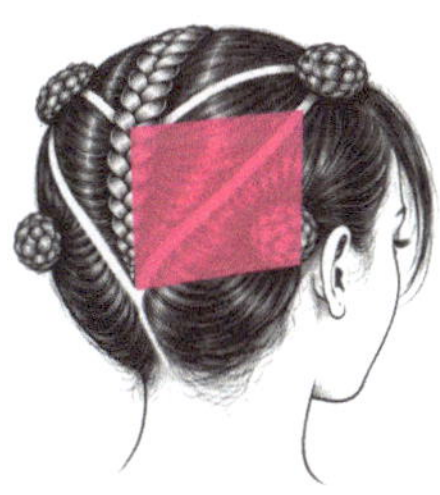

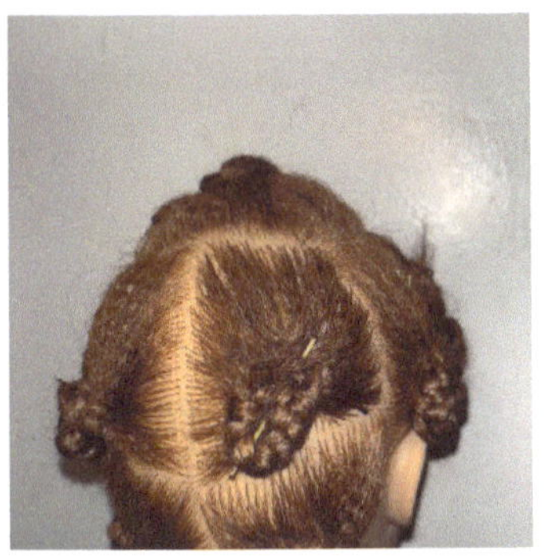
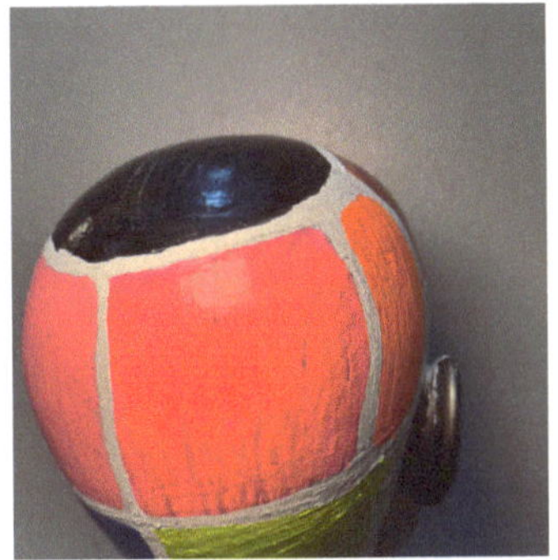

The **Back Right Region** outlines the space above the occipital bone and includes the visible upper back portion of the head. Hair in this region covers the neck and naturally falls straight downward, aligning with the spine.

When performing Scalp Manipulation, Detangling, or Hairstyling, position and guide the hair downward toward the center in alignment with the spine.

RECESSION LEFT

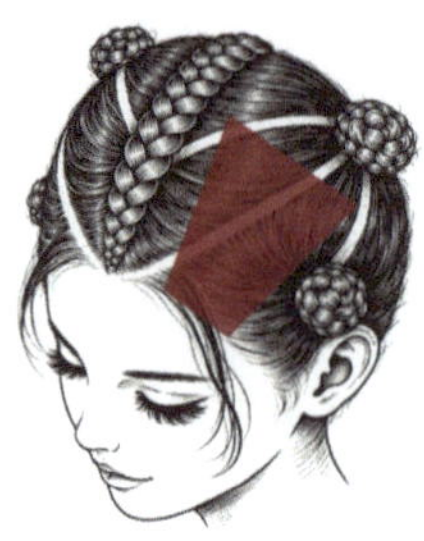

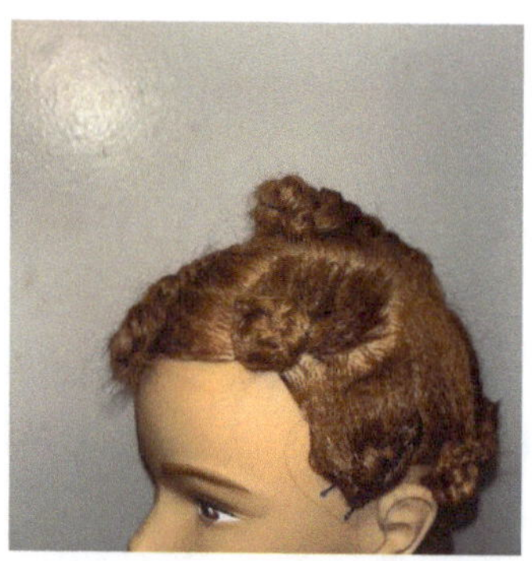
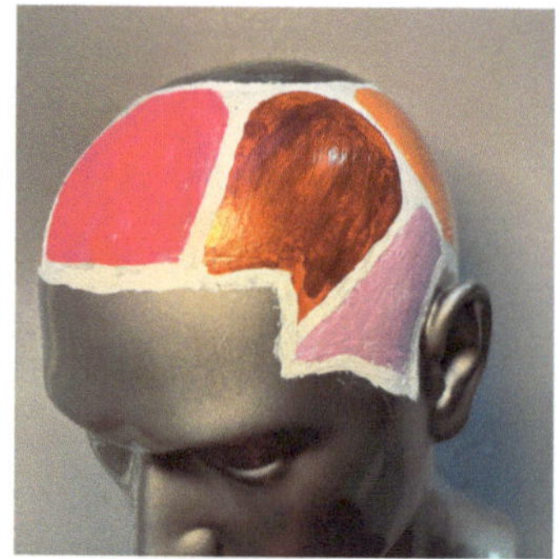

The **Recession Left region** highlights the natural curvature of the head, outlining the recessed area located above the Temporal region where the skull curves inward toward the forehead. Hair in this section provides coverage by connecting the Temporal region to the Forehead, guiding movement toward the face.

When performing Scalp Manipulation, Detangling, or Hairstyling, position and guide the hair toward the face and slightly downward.

RECESSION RIGHT

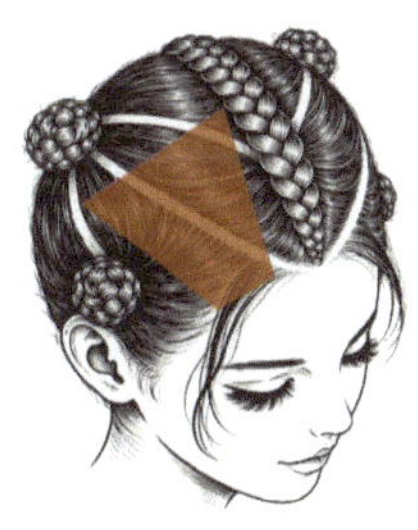

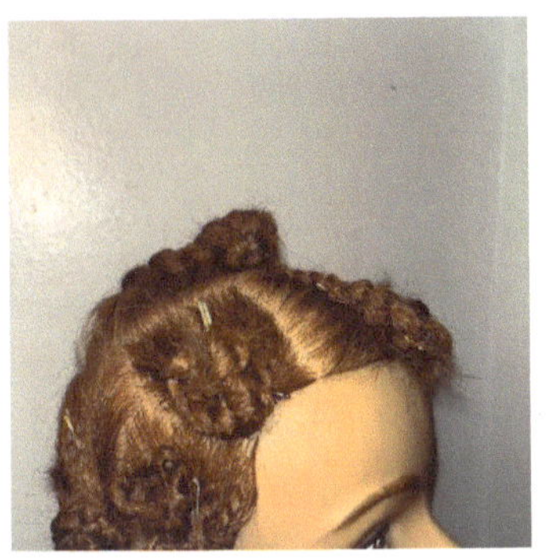
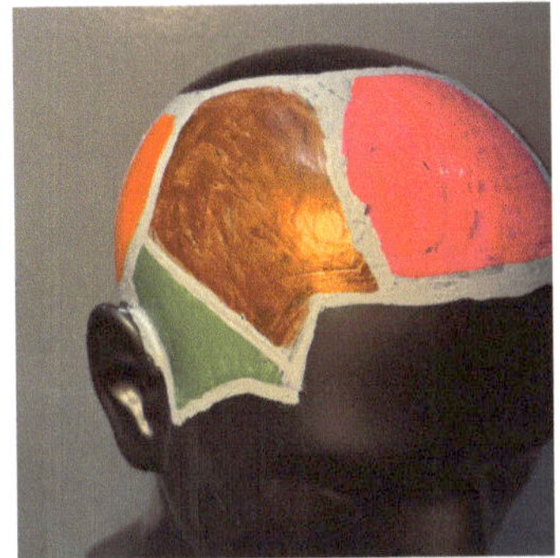

The **Recession Right region** highlights the natural curvature of the head, outlining the recessed area located above the Temporal region where the skull curves inward toward the forehead. Hair in this section provides coverage by connecting the Temporal region to the Forehead, guiding movement toward the face.

When performing Scalp Manipulation, Detangling, or Hairstyling, position and guide the hair toward the face and slightly downward.

FORGOTTEN ZONE LEFT

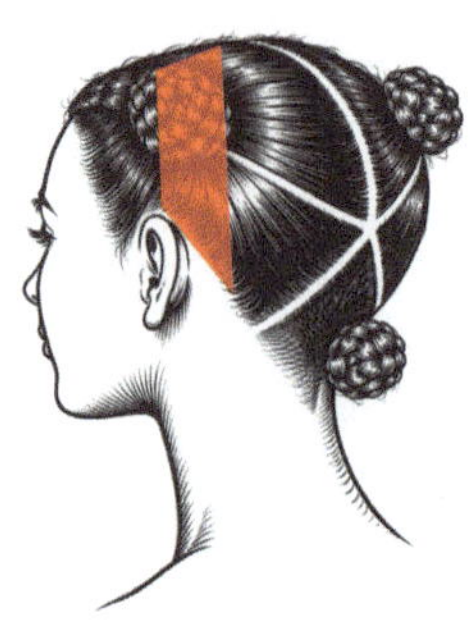

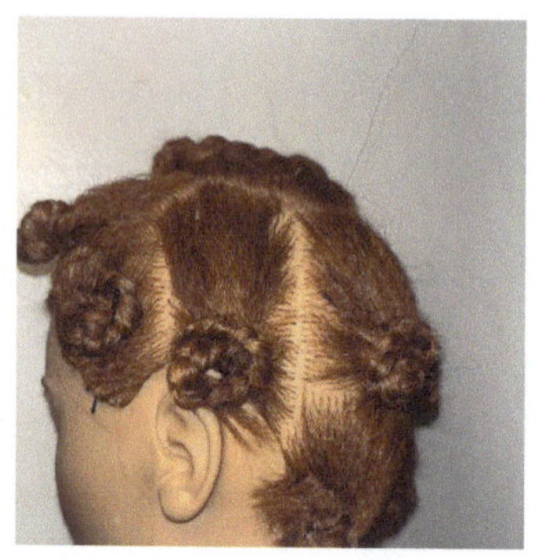
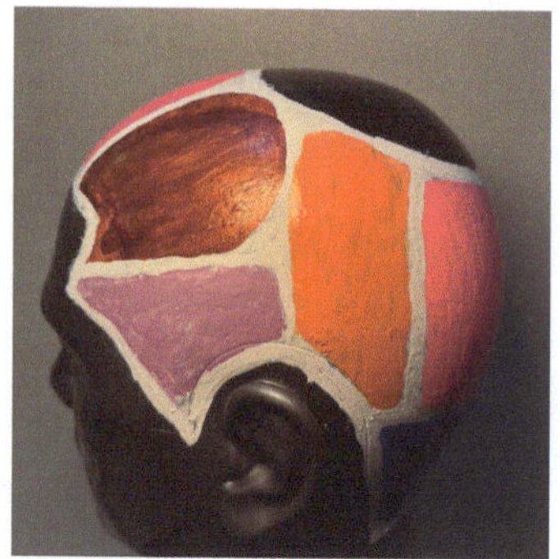

The **Forgotten Zone** highlights the transitional curvature of the head. This region connects the Temporal section to the Back section of the head. It sits partially above and slightly behind the ear, forming the bridge between the side and back regions. Hair in this area supports the natural blending between the Nape and Temporal zones, contributing to overall balance and coverage.

When performing Scalp Manipulation, Detangling & Hairstyling, position and guide the hair downward toward the ears and slightly diagonally toward the face.

FORGOTTEN ZONE RIGHT

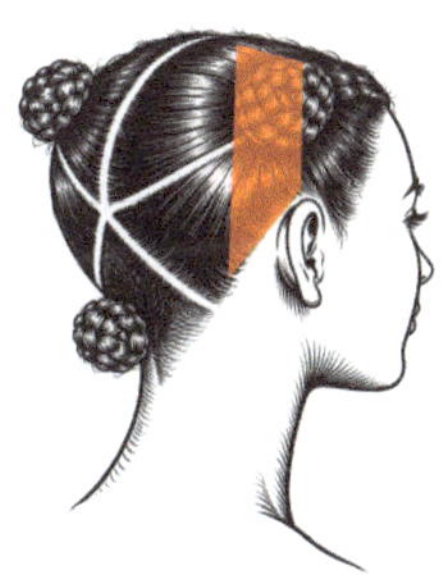

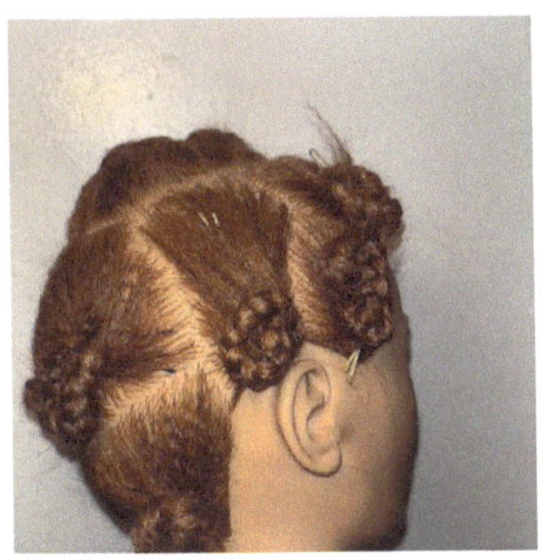 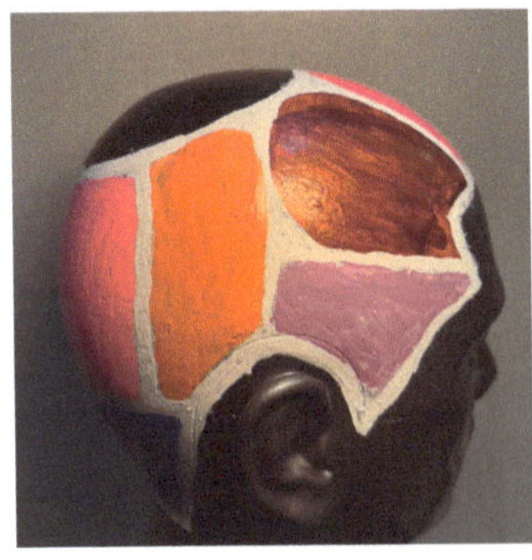

The **Forgotten Zone** highlights the transitional curvature of the head. This region connects the Temporal section to the Back section of the head. It sits partially above and slightly behind the ear, forming the bridge between the side and back regions. Hair in this area supports the natural blending between the Nape and Temporal zones, contributing to overall balance and coverage.

When performing Scalp Manipulation, Detangling & Hairstyling, position and guide the hair downward toward the ear and slightly diagonally toward the face.

FRINGE

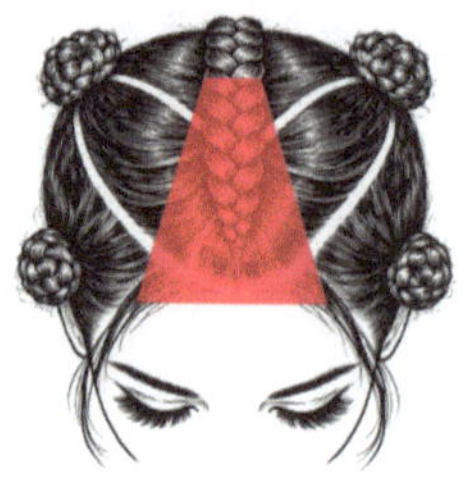

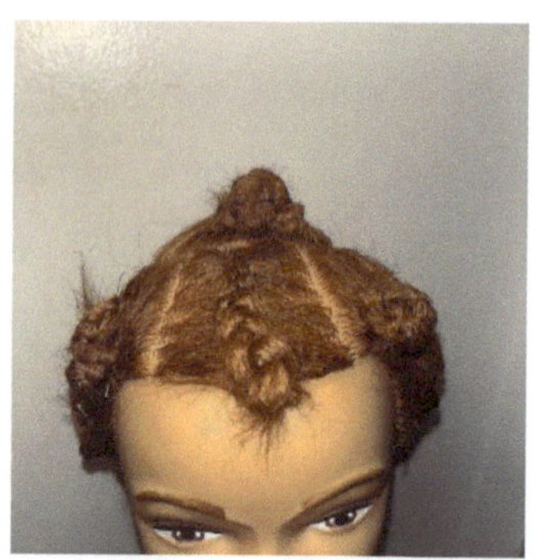
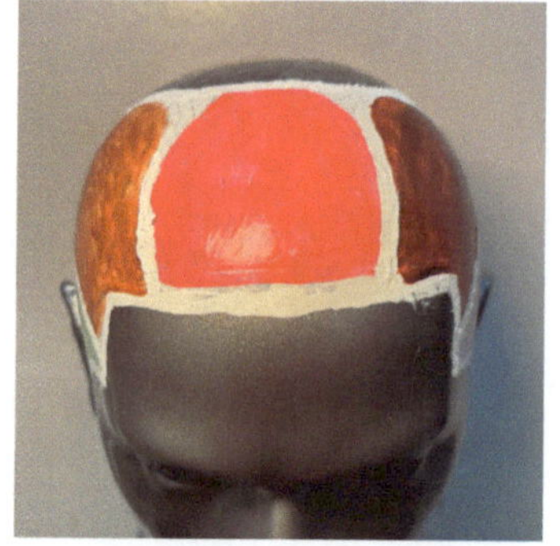

The **Fringe** is located in the frontal region of the head and is identified by the height of the brow, extending upward into the hairline. It forms a triangular shape that peaks at the highest point of the head, known as the Apex. This region provides primary coverage along the frontal perimeter and directs movement toward the face. It is commonly referred to as bangs.

When performing Scalp Manipulation, Detangling, or Hairstyling, position and guide the hair solely toward the face while respecting the natural hair parting.

CROWN

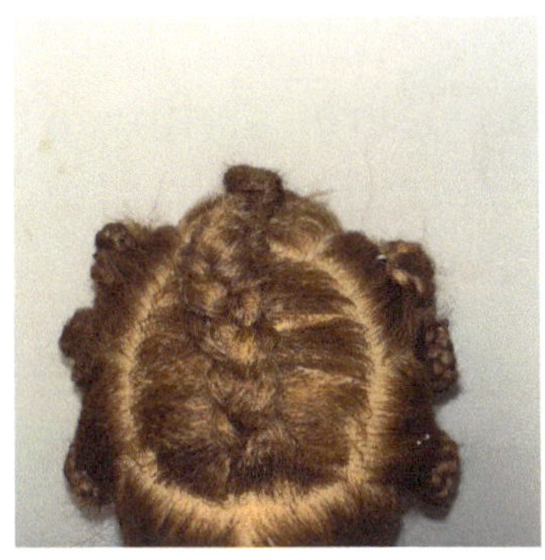 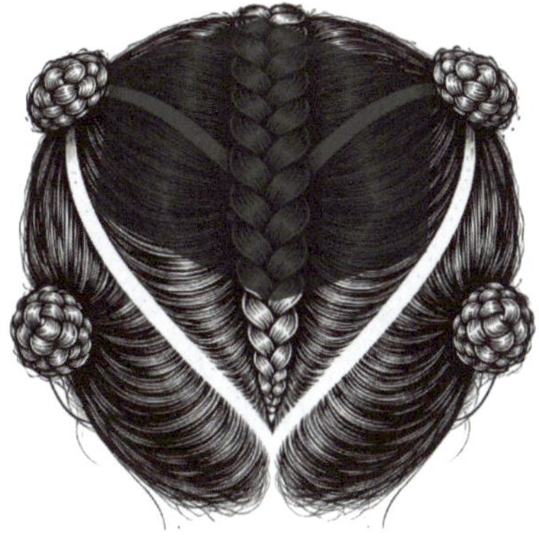 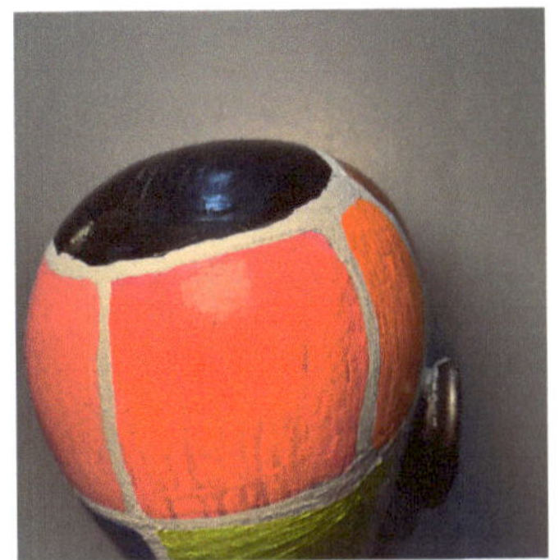

The Crown is the highest section of the head where the Apex exists. This region joins all major zones of the head and serves as the central balance point of the overall structure. Because it connects to the Fringe, Recession, Temporal, Forgotten, Back, and Nape regions, the Crown plays a critical role in controlling direction, movement, and coverage.

For structural control, the Crown can be divided into four working quadrants: front (toward the Fringe), right (connecting to the Temporal and Forgotten zones), left (mirroring the right side), and back (leading toward the Back and Nape regions).

Hair in this region naturally responds to growth patterns such as cowlicks and whorls. When performing Scalp Manipulation, Detangling & Hairstyling, position and guide the hair in a controlled downward circular motion or direct it from the center toward the intended section, respecting the natural growth pattern.

If you have made it this far, you have successfully navigated the entire human head. Note that there are complexities in all humans that differ from ours, but many things also connect us. Thank you for reading. I appreciate your optimism and hope I have brought you enlightenment. And yes, the information you just digested can be simplified as well...that is what Ponytails are for, lol. Now you know what is on the scalp **before** it goes into the ponytail.

Use this guide for Scalp Manipulation, Waving/360-degree styling, and Detangling. Protective styles: braids/twist-out/braid-out/bantu knots/locs & wiks, in addition to hairstyling sectioning, haircutting sectioning, hair color sectioning, chemical services, child & human friendly.

PICTURES AND REFERENCES

Mannequin One

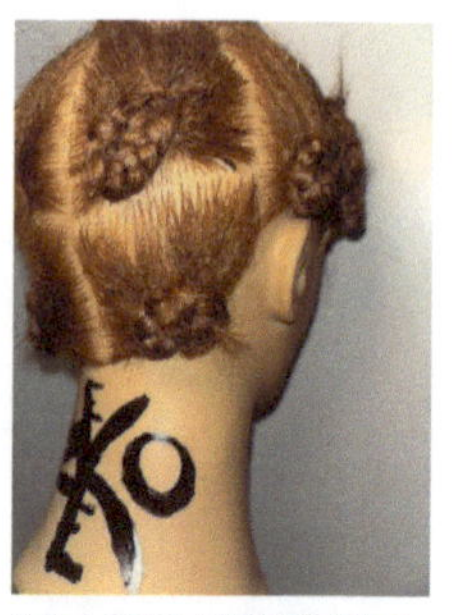

NAPE RIGHT

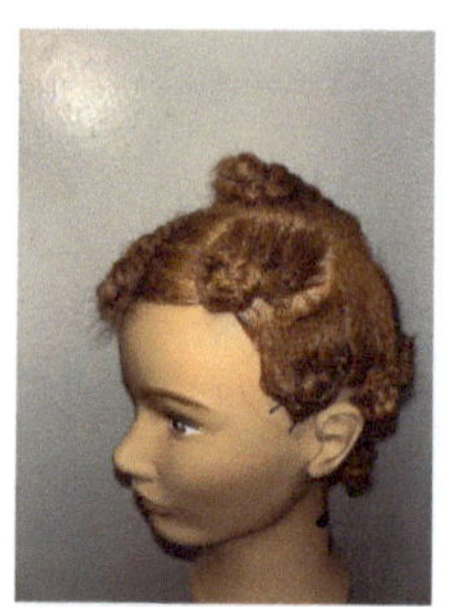

RECESSION LEFT

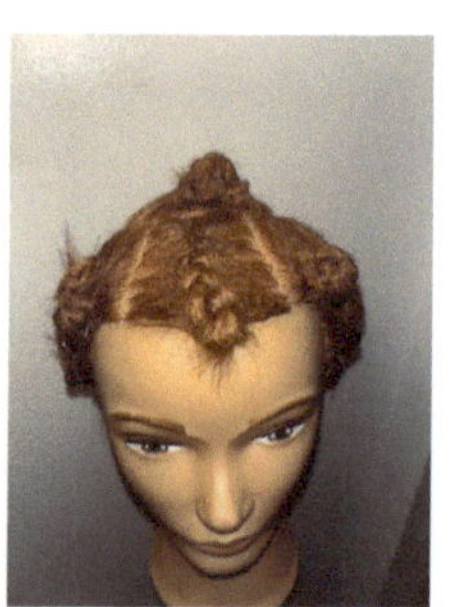

FRINGE

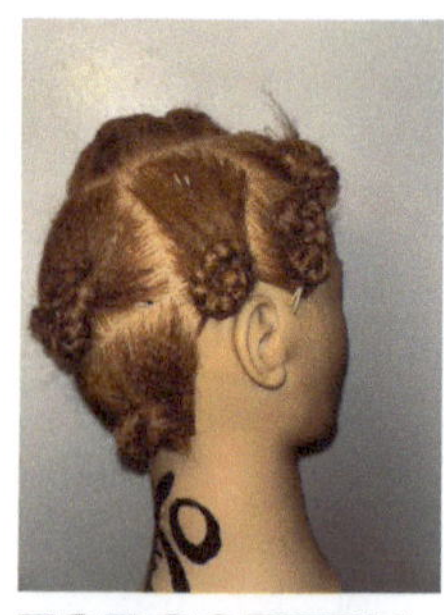

FORGOTTEN ZONE RIGHT

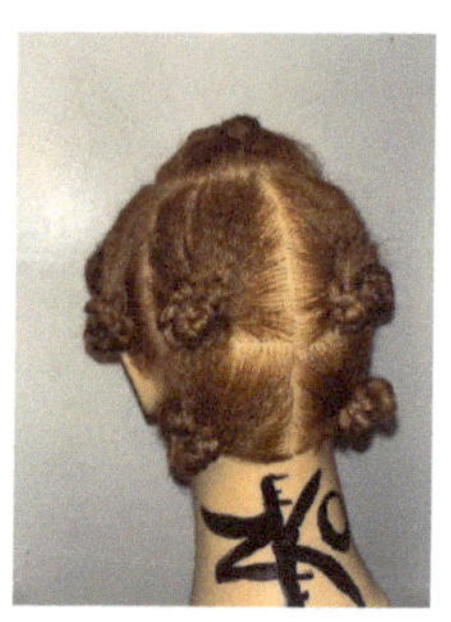

BACK LEFT

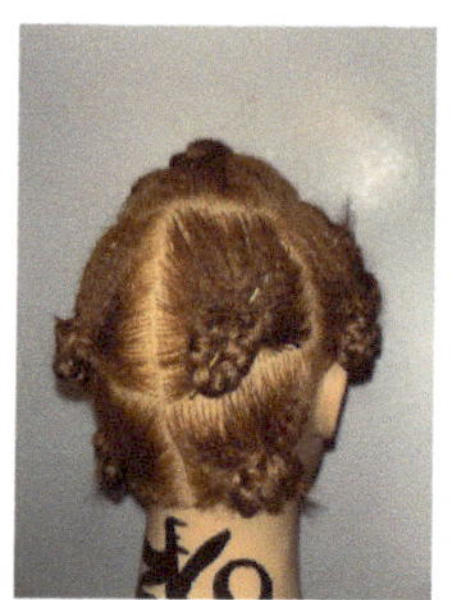

BACK RIGHT

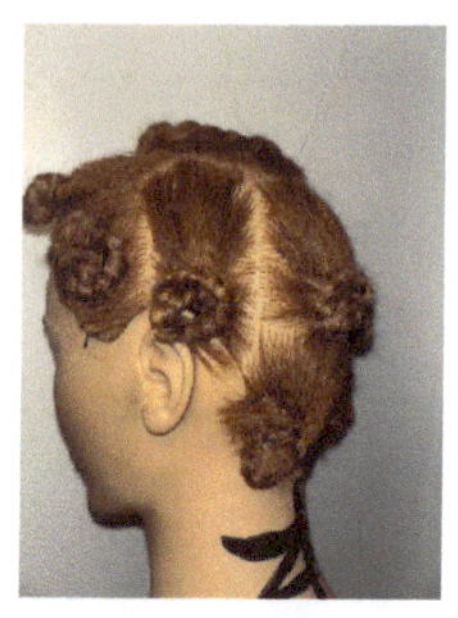

FORGOTTEN ZONE LEFT

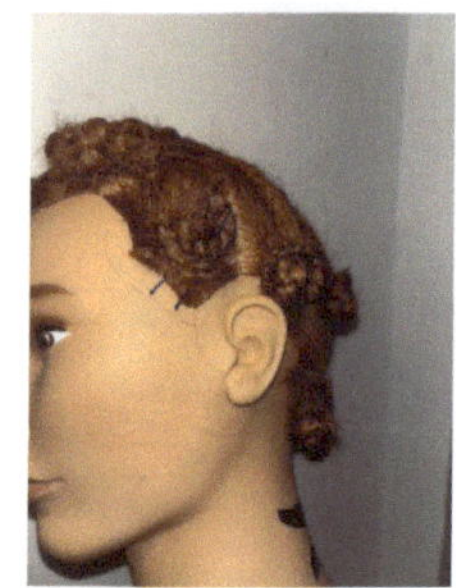

TEMPORAL LEFT

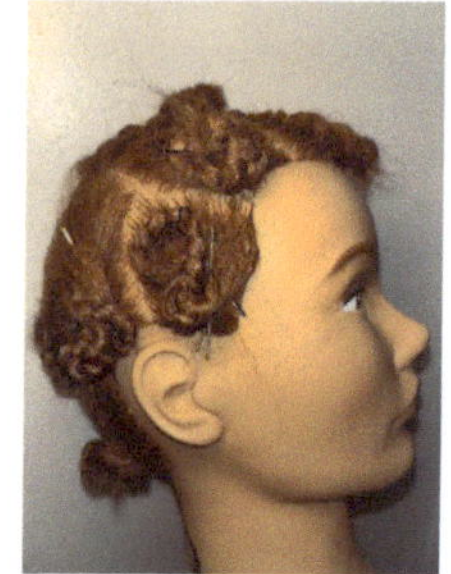

TEMPORAL RIGHT

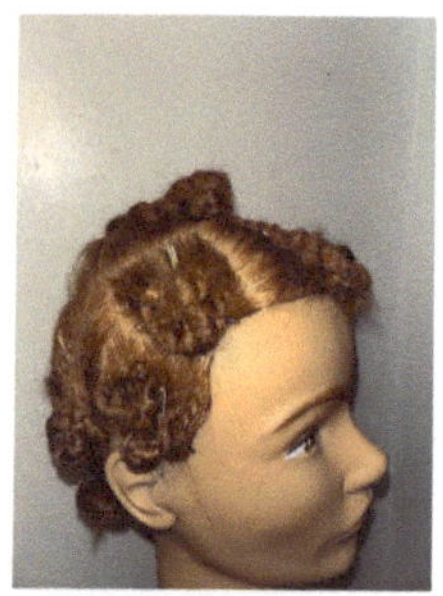

RECESSION RIGHT

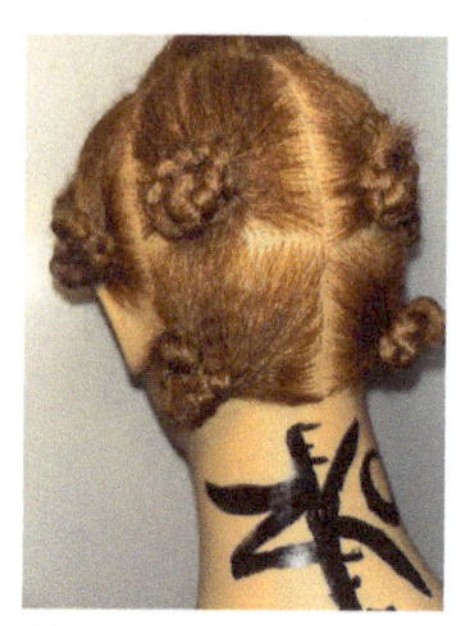

NAPE LEFT

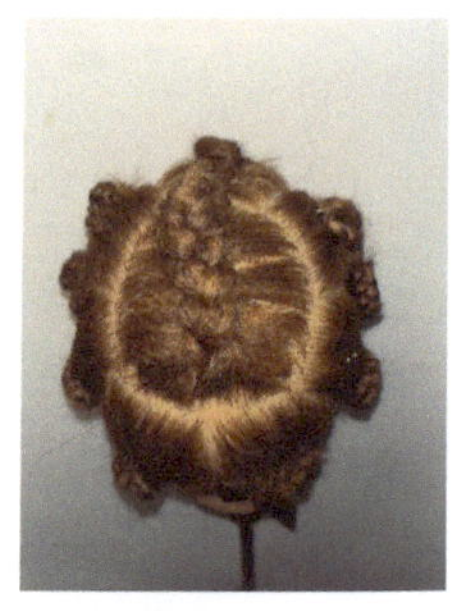

CROWN

Mannequin Two

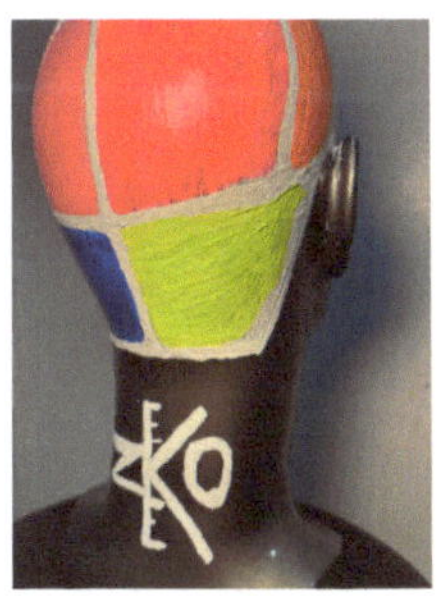

NAPE RIGHT

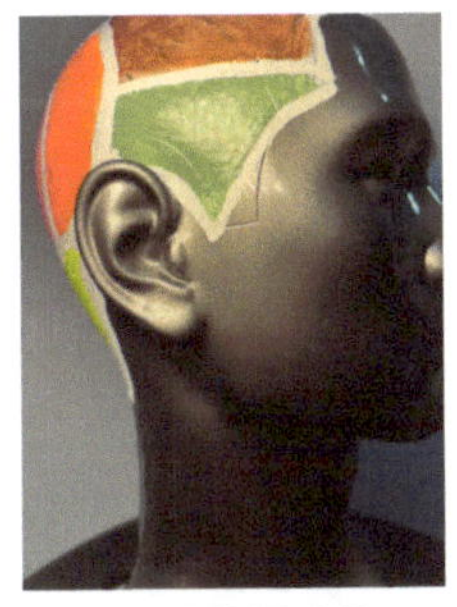

TEMPORAL RIGHT

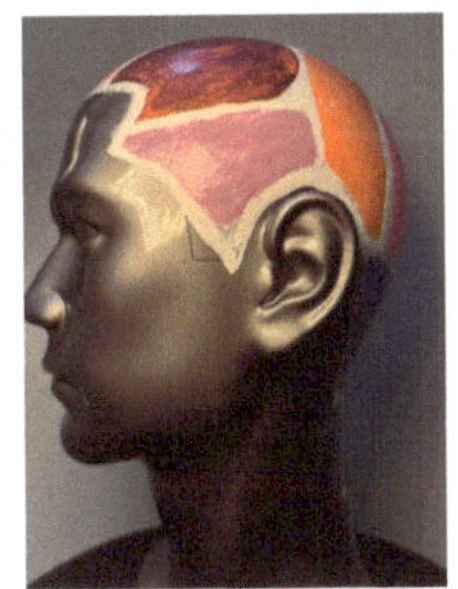

TEMPORAL LEFT

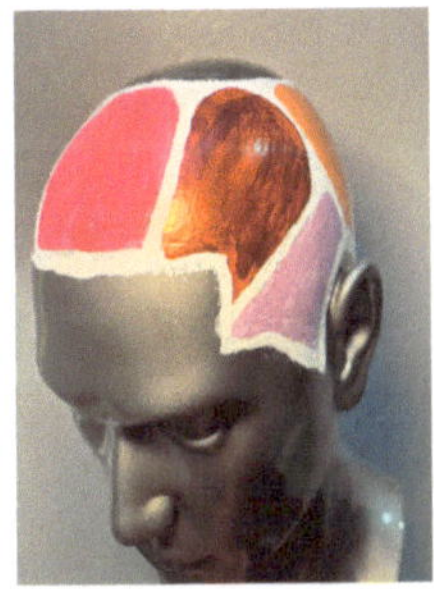

RECESSION LEFT

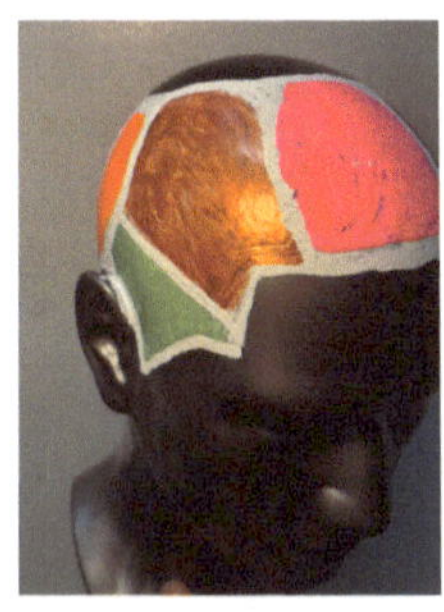

RECESSION RIGHT

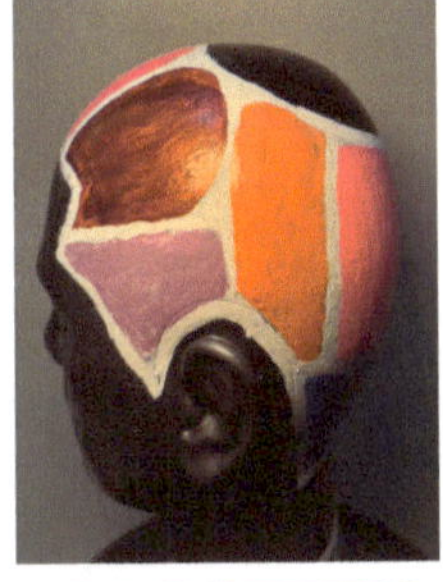

FORGOTTEN ZONE LEFT

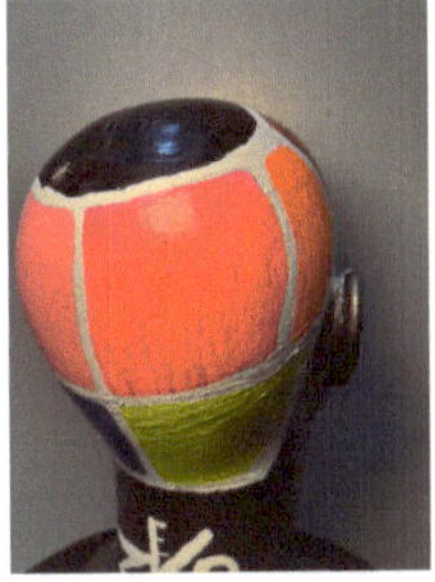

BACK RIGHT

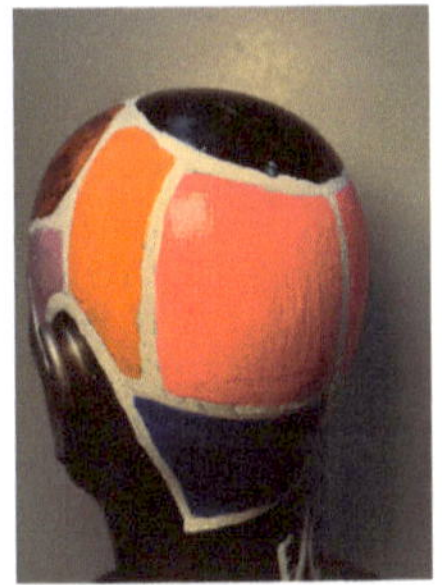

BACK LEFT

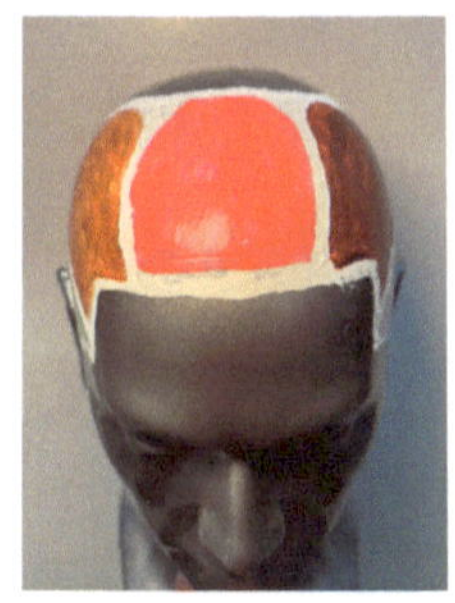

FRINGE

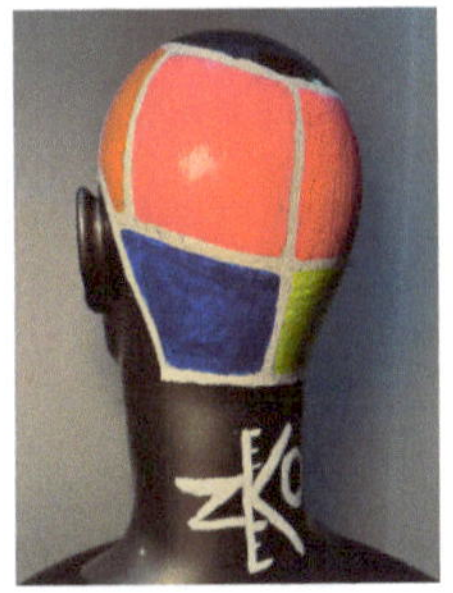

NAPE LEFT

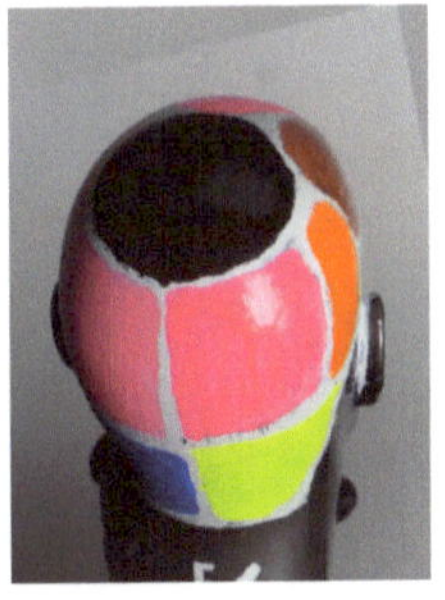

CROWN

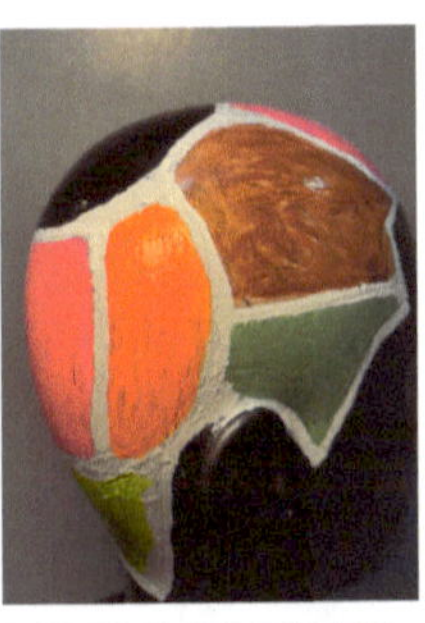

FORGOTTEN ZONE RIGHT

Illustrations

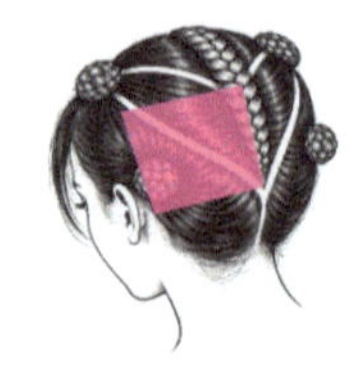

BACK LEFT

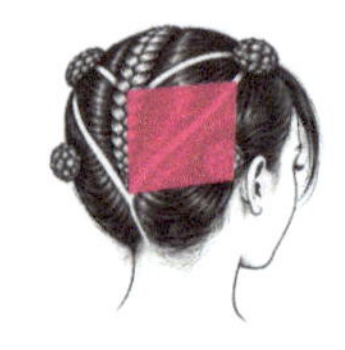

BACK RIGHT

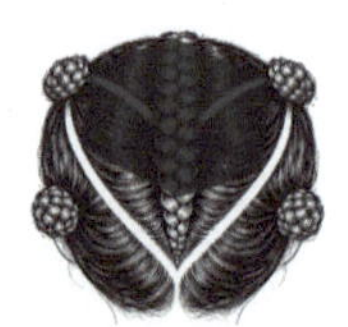

CROWN

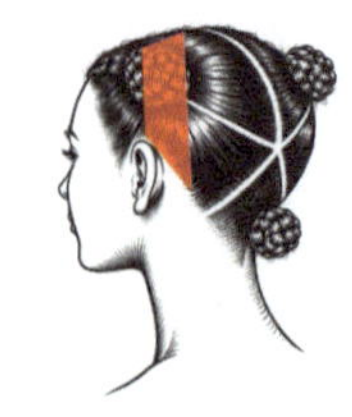

FORGOTTEN ZONE LEFT

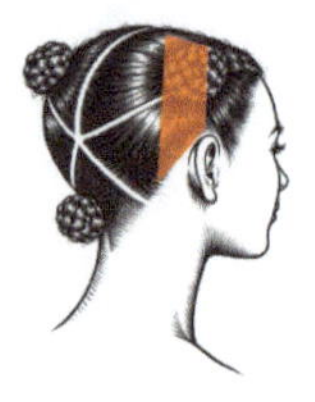

FORGOTTEN ZONE RIGHT

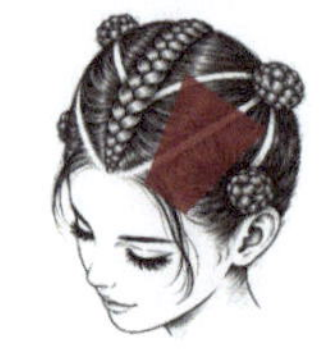

RECESSION LEFT

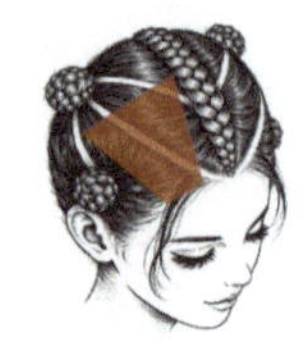

RECESSION RIGHT

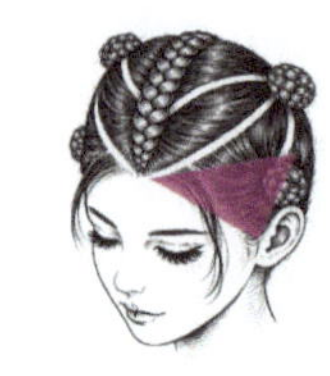

TEMPORAL LEFT

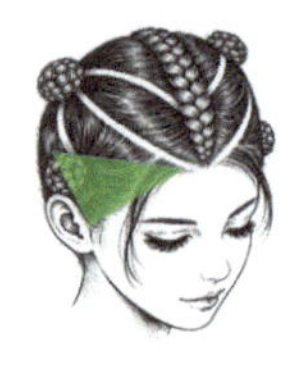

TEMPORAL RIGHT

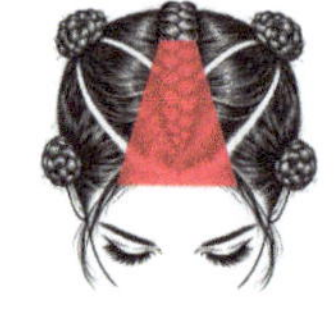

FRINGE

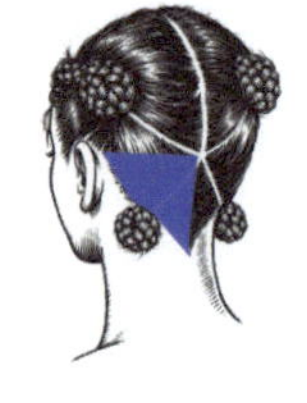

NAPE LEFT

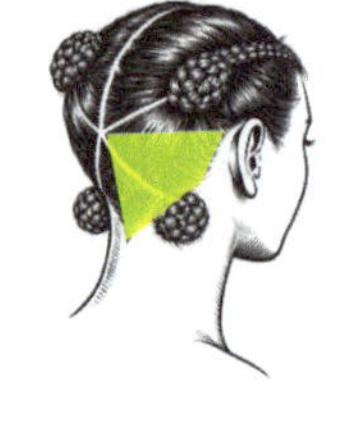

NAPE RIGHT